Building Practice Revenue
A Guide to Developing New Services

Bruce A. Johnson, JD, MPA

Darrell L. Schryver, DPA

Daniel P Stech MBA

Medical Group
Management
Association

Medical Group Management Association
104 Inverness Terrace East
Englewood, CO   80112
877.275.6462
Web site: www.mgma.com

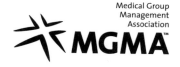

Medical Group
Management
Association

Medical Group Management (MGMA) publications are intended to provide current and accurate information and are designed to assist readers in becoming more familiar with the subject matter covered. Such publications are distributed with the understanding that MGMA does not render any legal, accounting or other professional advice that may be construed as specifically applicable to individual situations. No representations or warranties are made concerning the application of legal or other principles discussed by the authors to any specific factual situation, nor is any prediction made concerning how any particular judge, government official, or other person will interpret or apply such principles. Specific factual situations should be discussed with professional advisors.

Cover photo courtesy of Photodisc

Item #6073

Copyright © 2003 Medical Group Management Association

ISBN 1-56829-229-5

Printed in the United States of America

10 9 8 7 6 5 4 3 2 1

Contents

List of Figures and Tables

Notes and Checklists

Acknowledgments

The authors would like to recognize the contribution of a select group of practice administrators who assisted in compiling data for this publication. They include: Jean G. Becker, Mary A. Bechler, FACMPE, Robin J. Brown, CMPE, and Suzette Jaskie, MBA.

Bruce A. Johnson, JD, MPA

Bruce Johnson is special counsel, Faegre & Benson, LLP and a consultant with the MGMA Health Care Consulting Group. He brings over 15 years of health care-related legal and management experience to his clients in medical group practices, faculty practice plans, hospitals integrated systems and others. Bruce is an expert on the planning, development and implementation of new business service lines, including wholly-owned and joint venture diagnostic imaging, ambulatory surgical and other ancillary service ventures. His law practice focuses on the application of the federal physician self-referral or "Stark" law, antikickback, Medicare reimbursement, tax-exempt organization and related legal issues to medical practice business activities. A frequent national speaker on a variety of topics, he is the author of three books and numerous articles on health care-related topics, and is the developer and manager of MGMA's StarkCompliance Solutions web-based product (www.starkcompliance.com). He received a juris doctor degree from the University of Colorado School of Law and a master's degree in public administration from The Ohio State University.

Darrell L. Schryver, DPA

Darrell L. Schryver, DPA, is a principal consultant with the MGMA Health Care Consulting Group and a faculty member for the ACMPE Management Education and Development (MED) Series. Prior to joining MGMA, Darrell was a professor of Health Care Management/Economics at Metropolitan State College of Denver where he taught upper division courses in health care economics, finance, managed care, management issues and integrated delivery system development. His background spans over 30 years of health care management where he held senior executive positions in hospitals, single and multispecialty group practices and with a national health care consulting firm. He is a frequent national lecturer and contributing author to more than 50 articles in leading health care journals and publications. He is also a contributor to three health care textbooks and is the editor of the MGMA Assessment Manual for Medical Groups. Darrell received a master's degree in business administration from Sul Ross University and a doctorate in public administration with a concentration in health care economics from Nova Southeastern University.

Daniel P. Stech, MBA

Daniel P. Stech has been the director of the MGMA Survey Operations Department since March 2001. He began his career with MGMA in 1995 as a state health policy analyst, and served as director of the MGMA Health Care Consulting Group from 1997 to 2001. Prior to joining the MGMA staff, Dan held various legislative staff positions with U.S. Representative Earl Hutto where he specialized in issues related to health system reform, regulation and reimbursement. He blends his knowledge of health policy and his experience in health business to help lead MGMA's survey activity and support a variety of association initiatives. Dan serves as a member and industry resource on medical practice trends and business improvement through data analysis and the application of benchmarks. He received a master of business administration degree from Marymount University in Arlington, VA, and is currently a Nominee in the American College of Medical Practice Executives.

Understanding the Issue and the Opportunity

Reimbursement for physician and other professional services under Medicare Part B increased an anemic 1.6% in 2003, and that increase only occurred after considerable outcry by the physician community and congressional action. Estimates of future trends indicate that this respite from reimbursement cuts will likely be short-lived, as Medicare Part B reimbursement is projected to decrease in the years ahead. And because commercial reimbursement levels are increasingly benchmarked to Medicare rates, future reimbursement cuts will not be limited to public payers. In the face of these and other external challenges, physicians, medical groups and group practice administrators are exploring ways to expand or diversify their existing revenue streams.

This book is designed to outline ideas, opportunities and practical guidance regarding revenue diversification and ancillary service opportunities. It is intended to provide information and tools on a number of specific questions and themes.

Our orientation in this resource is both general and specific. We focus much of our attention on the application of sound business concepts to ancillary service and other revenue diversification strategies. We apply and illustrate these general concepts through case studies that summarize the experiences of successful medical groups in developing new service lines. These examples are presented in the context of our broader discussion on how medical groups should systematically assess and develop new business opportunities, along with potential structural alternatives.

With this book, you'll be able to answer these questions:

1. What benefits and challenges might be associated with various revenue diversification options such as ancillary and other new services for any medical group practice?

2. How might a medical group, its physicians and administrative leadership approach the development and implementation of successful ancillary service and other revenue diversification strategies?

3. What alternative structural models might be considered, and what legal issues and opportunities will be relevant to proposed revenue opportunities?

4. What other resources and tools can medical groups use to guide their efforts in a systematic and structured way?

Consistent with our emphasis on highlighting ideas and opportunities, Chapter 2 reviews some of the facts and potential benefits of revenue-stream diversification. The data in this chapter illustrate the outcome of decisions made by medical groups, so we present only a partial picture of the potential financial opportunities available to medical practices today. The range of potentially profitable ancillary service or new business lines—collectively referred to as revenue opportunities—will continue to change in the years ahead. But just as paying attention to billings, collections and practice operating costs is essential to the short- and long-term financial viability of a medical group, this chapter demonstrates how close consideration of new services, relationships and a willingness to think "outside the box" can yield significant returns.

Chapter 3 presents an analytical approach to assessing revenue opportunities. In today's challenging health care delivery and reimbursement environments, medical practices frequently consider numerous "good ideas" for increasing practice profits, conserving costs and enhancing the bottom line. However, without a structured and rational approach to analysis, decision making and the implementation of new revenue opportunities, a practice risks missing out on useful opportunities or incurring financial loss for poor decisions or faulty implementation. We outline an analytical approach that can assist a practice in choosing and developing a revenue-producing venture integrated into the practice's broader business strategy.

The complex requirements of today's legal and regulatory environments have significant implications for any number of potential revenue opportunities. Chapter 4 reviews some of the major legal issues affecting medical group revenue diversification strategies and outlines potential structural models that may be available in many jurisdictions. Readers should keep in mind that a book of this nature can provide only a general, high-level review of such issues and the health care legal environment is subject to almost constant change. Therefore, the development and implementation of a legally compliant revenue diversification strategy will require the assistance of health care legal counsel. Nevertheless, Chapter 4 and the appendixes provide ideas, examples of structural alternatives and checklists that can help guide the reader through the intricate health care legal and regulatory landscape.

The strategies outlined here are largely presented for objective guidance and tools to help promote medical practice success. Of course, success in a medical group depends on numerous factors that extend beyond issues of financial profitability. Other success fundamentals must always serve as the foundation for any revenue diversification or ancillary service venture, including the core obligations of medical business outlined below.

The Fundamental Obligations of Medical Business

- Medically appropriate services consistent with the needs of patient care;

- Furnished by personnel with appropriate training, skills and professional competence; and

- Provided in compliance with applicable laws and rules.

These requirements serve as a tripod upon which the business and operational plans for any ancillary service or other revenue opportunity must rest. Weaknesses or defects in any one of these areas will risk unbalancing the revenue diversification strategy business model, therefore undermining prospects for success.

Know the Basics

- Reimbursement rates for both Medicare and commercial insurers are not expected to increase in the foreseeable future.

- Developing new revenue requires medical organizations to think creatively and examine nontraditional business activities.

- Thorough business planning is critical to the successful creation of new revenue-producing activities.

- Revenue diversification strategies have legal and regulatory implications.

- Satisfying medical business fundamentals is essential to any new business activity.

Why do Revenue Opportunities Matter?
Basic Facts and Considerations

The need for new sources of revenue in medical groups is based on the harsh realities of medicine today. Reimbursement is generally declining while operating costs continue to rise.

Figure 2.1 on the following page summarizes the projected trends in Medicare reimbursement over the next few years. It illustrates projected changes in Part B reimbursement from federal health care payers as of March 2003. And although private-pay reimbursement differs from Medicare reimbursement levels, the underlying trends in Medicare nevertheless have implications for private-payer reimbursement levels.

Figure 2.1

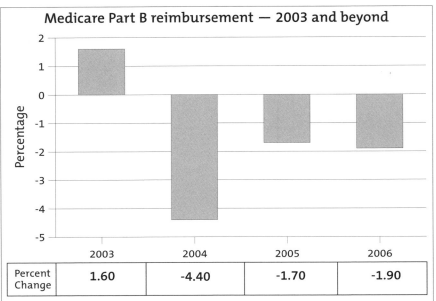

Medicare Part B reimbursement — 2003 and beyond

	2003	2004	2005	2006
Percent Change	1.60	-4.40	-1.70	-1.90

Projected percentage rate of change in Medicare Part B reimbursement, 2003-2006
Source: *2003 Annual Report of the Boards of Trustees of the Federal Hospital Insurance and Federal Supplemental Medical Insurance Trust Funds*, March 17, 2003.

Physicians commonly hold the view that operating costs — or overhead — continues to increase. Figure 2.2 presents historic information related to medical practice operating costs expressed as a percentage of net medical revenues for multispecialty practices. It demonstrates that over the past 15 years, medical practice costs as a percentage of practice revenues have increased. The perception of increasing overhead tends to be enhanced due to a variety of factors, including declining reimbursement levels, additional compliance burdens, managed care and increased complexity. In bottom-line terms, Figure 2.2 demonstrates that medical practice challenges have obvious implications for profits and the income levels of physicians, other providers and staff.

Figure 2.2

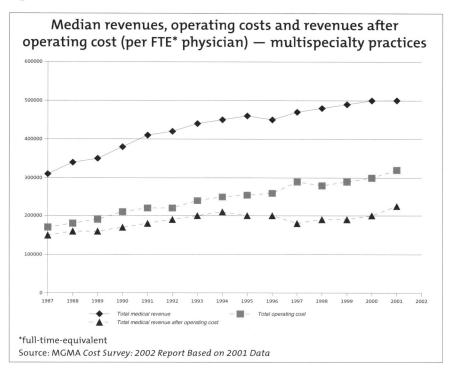

Median revenues, operating costs and revenues after operating cost (per FTE* physician) — multispecialty practices

Legend:
◆ Total medical revenue
■ Total operating cost
▲ Total medical revenue after operating cost

*full-time-equivalent
Source: MGMA *Cost Survey: 2002 Report Based on 2001 Data*

Is there hope? In the face of declining reimbursement and increasing costs, must medical practices, their physicians, providers and staff work ever harder or face stagnant or declining levels of compensation? Experience demonstrates that even in the complex world of health care, working "smarter" is a viable option to sustaining — if not improving — a practice's bottom line. And among the working-smarter strategies are those that focus on the development of new sources of income through revenue-stream diversification and ancillary service development.

Potential Revenue Opportunities

Medical groups today are considering and developing numerous potential revenue opportunities, including:

- Diagnostic imaging services (e.g., MRI, nuclear imaging, dexascan);

- In-office catherization laboratories and endoscopy suites;

- Procedures, products and services consistent with provider specialties and clinically indicated, such as new drug treatments and therapies (e.g., botox and other cosmetic services), new procedures and treatment modalities (e.g., bariatric surgery, laser procedures);

- Investments in ambulatory surgery centers and specialty hospitals; and

- Alternative and complementary treatment therapies and treatment modalities (e.g., acupuncture, psychological services) as part of or in conjunction with the medical practice's core functions.

The rapid change in health care most likely means that the range of revenue opportunities that medical practices pursue today may *not* constitute the complement of services they will provide or will profit from tomorrow. But today's experiences can provide information for the future, while helping practices understand the relevant factors to performance and success.

Available data clearly indicate that better-performing medical groups tend to differ from others in any number of areas, most notably the services they provide and the manner in which they seize opportunities to profit from medically appropriate services.

Figure 2.3

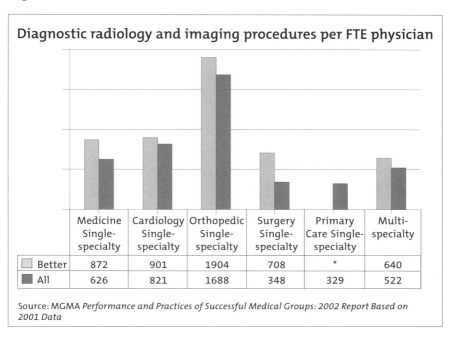

Diagnostic radiology and imaging procedures per FTE physician

	Medicine Single-specialty	Cardiology Single-specialty	Orthopedic Single-specialty	Surgery Single-specialty	Primary Care Single-specialty	Multi-specialty
Better	872	901	1904	708	*	640
All	626	821	1688	348	329	522

Source: MGMA *Performance and Practices of Successful Medical Groups: 2002 Report Based on 2001 Data*

Figure 2.3 presents data relating to the number of diagnostic radiology and imaging procedures per full-time-equivalent (FTE) physician in better-performing and single-specialty medical groups as of 2001. Better-performing medical groups tend to have higher volumes of procedures per physician, which translates into increased profitability.

Figure 2.4

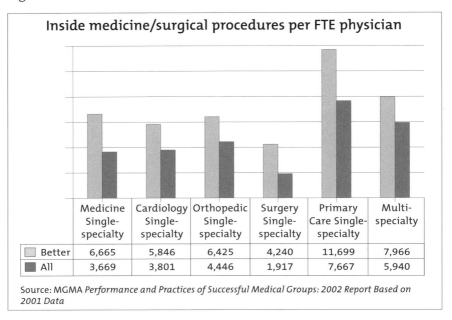

Inside medicine/surgical procedures per FTE physician

	Medicine Single-specialty	Cardiology Single-specialty	Orthopedic Single-specialty	Surgery Single-specialty	Primary Care Single-specialty	Multi-specialty
Better	6,665	5,846	6,425	4,240	11,699	7,966
All	3,669	3,801	4,446	1,917	7,667	5,940

Source: MGMA *Performance and Practices of Successful Medical Groups: 2002 Report Based on 2001 Data*

Figure 2.4 presents a similar story, but with respect to medicine and surgical procedures per FTE physician performed inside the practice. Here too, better performers tend to do more or provide more services within their practices compared with the average medical group.

Figure 2.5

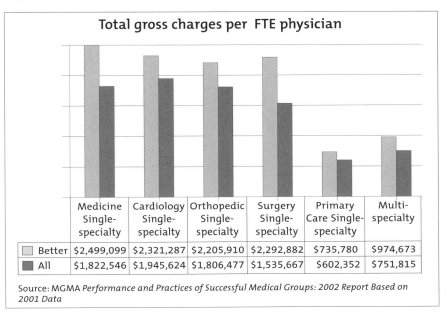

	Medicine Single-specialty	Cardiology Single-specialty	Orthopedic Single-specialty	Surgery Single-specialty	Primary Care Single-specialty	Multi-specialty
Better	$2,499,099	$2,321,287	$2,205,910	$2,292,882	$735,780	$974,673
All	$1,822,546	$1,945,624	$1,806,477	$1,535,667	$602,352	$751,815

Source: MGMA *Performance and Practices of Successful Medical Groups: 2002 Report Based on 2001 Data*

Figure 2.5 presents the economic payoff of these services in the form of higher gross charges, and therefore, opportunities for greater amounts of cash per FTE physician.

These data illustrate how efforts by better-performing medical groups to enhance or optimize the services that are furnished by and through the practice can yield positive dividends. These groups have, in many instances, worked proactively to develop diagnostic services that can be furnished through the medical practice's offices. Many such groups have also developed surgical suites to furnish minor and/or elective outpatient surgical procedures.

But not every surgical procedure can or should be furnished through the medical group. Certain services can and should be furnished through ambulatory surgical centers (ASCs) or hospital facilities equipped for more complex surgical operations cases. Here, too, the data reveal a significant difference between those organizations that work to furnish more services in-house and those that do not.

Figure 2.6 shows comparative data for orthopedic practices with or without a wholly owned ambulatory surgical center. Of course, this figure only presents the differences in bottom-line financial terms. Practices that have ASCs within their service-delivery arsenal will also commonly identify less tangible but still significant benefits. These include enhanced patient convenience, enhanced physician efficiency and improvements in quality because the ASC and its staff can specialize in a defined subset of surgical procedures.

Figure 2.6

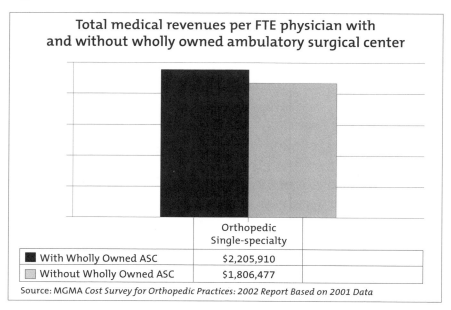

Total medical revenues per FTE physician with and without wholly owned ambulatory surgical center

	Orthopedic Single-specialty	
■ With Wholly Owned ASC	$2,205,910	
□ Without Wholly Owned ASC	$1,806,477	

Source: MGMA *Cost Survey for Orthopedic Practices: 2002 Report Based on 2001 Data*

In light of reimbursement and other challenges that will most likely confront medical practices and their physicians for the foreseeable future, these and other data highlight a number of differences between better-performing medical groups and their peers. The factors of profitability in medical groups, like any other business, will continue to be essential. Practices must continue to focus on both revenues and expenses of the clinical enterprise. Yet because practice operating costs are, under even the best of scenarios, likely to remain stable (if not increase), successful groups must pay equal attention to optimizing and diversifying the revenue stream.

To that end, better-performing medical groups commonly focus on three core activities:

1. **Enhancing the efficiency and volume of services per unit of medical practice fixed cost.** Fixed or fixed variable costs comprise upwards of 60%-80% of the typical medical practice's cost structure. Successful groups optimize the services furnished through the use of that fixed cost structure. This includes expanding hours, developing creative patient scheduling processes and finding the best means of using fixed resources, such as facilities and equipment.

2. **Identifying outsourced services that can be brought in-house or otherwise furnished under the practice's control.** Groups considering MRI and other diagnostic services frequently determine that significant numbers of procedures are furnished as a result of group referrals to other providers, including local hospitals and third-party vendors. They commonly find that the group's existing volume will support an in-house diagnostic effort, while helping to supplement the practice's existing revenue base.

3. **Including the idea of revenue diversification and the structured consideration of potential revenue opportunities as part of the medical group's overall business model and strategy.** Better-performing medical groups recognize that the best long-term strategy is one that involves a nearly constant quest for opportunities and positive change. Better-performing groups are typically learning organizations in which the providers and staff are encouraged to consider new ideas and question existing practices. Those ideas will commonly relate to new means to accomplish the practice's mission, such as innovative operational practices and creative staffing models. They'll also often involve consideration of more fundamental issues, including the practice's core and complementary service lines.

Know the Basics

Essential elements of any practice's long-term success include:

- Expanding and diversifying the practice's revenue stream;

- Reconsidering the ways and practices of the past; and

- An ability and willingness to think "outside of the box."

As practice operating costs continue to escalate in the face of declining or stagnant reimbursement, practices that fail to consider new business models, service lines and revenue opportunities risk stagnation, reduced income levels and even potential business failure in the years ahead.

An Analytical Approach to Assessing Revenue Diversification Opportunities

Developing new ancillary business activities has great appeal from a revenue standpoint and may even seem simple to more progressive medical groups. However, do not underestimate the operational, financial and legal requirements of implementation. Moreover, the viability of new services may rest as much upon environmental factors as upon the operational prowess of the group. A careful examination of all of these issues and the level of organizational commitment is imperative. This chapter provides an approach to thorough business planning in connection with revenue diversification.

From an administrative perspective, a medical practice's observation of fundamental business principles will drive its overall performance and success. While volumes can and have been written on effective business practices, many successful medical groups demonstrate adherence to a clear vision of their future, an ability to change with their environment and an understanding that medical groups must function as a business.

Got to have these:

- **Shared vision** — all group members must share a desire to diversify and grow.

- **Ability to adapt to environmental changes** — denial and resistance are the first two reactions to change. Groups need to identify opportunities presented by environmental change instead of focusing on potential losses.

- **Knowledge that medicine is business** — the emotional elements of health care must be balanced with objective business thinking and decision making.

Business analytical processes such as feasibility assessments, comparative analyses, opportunity cost assessment and zero-base budgeting are not only important principles of a successful practice administrator's intellectual repertoire, but their appropriate application may determine a medical group's future viability.

The operating environment for medical groups today is characterized by declining reimbursement, escalating costs, economic uncertainty, rapid change and the ever-increasing encroachment of government and regulations. Many groups attempt to maintain income and profitability by seeing more patients or doing more surgery. While appropriate in some instances, these strategies may themselves risk the future viability of the practice due to provider burnout, poor patient satisfaction and other unintended consequences.

Yet as illustrated in Chapter 2, many medical groups and their administrative leadership recognize the importance of "working smarter" in connection with the medical practice's care delivery model and business strategy. These organizations commonly have administrative, physician and other leadership that are more willing to consider and undertake strategic initiatives that promote change and enhance revenues, increase profitability and the group's overall economic success. Profitable medical groups tend to accept and incorporate the fundamental principles referenced above into their core operating strategies.

Inclusive Assessment Process Model. Experience in health care, as in other businesses and industries, suggests that only rarely will the "great idea" automatically lead to a successful product or business. Even the best concepts typically require close consideration and planning to refine ideas into a workable product, taking into account the cost of production, marketing and distribution strategies and all the details essential to moving from concept to reality.

Because medical practices are businesses, these same truths exist with any new business activity. Clearly, some revenue diversification strategies will constitute "no-brainers" for the practice and its providers in terms of financial costs and associated benefits. The furnishing of an additional service that is merely an incremental extension of current offerings will frequently fall into such a category.

Yet even here, as with other, more elaborate opportunities, the consideration of a new service line should be incorporated into an overall strategy that structures the assessment and implementation process into separate phases or processes that build on each other and are expressed in a business plan. The four phases central to any revenue diversification opportunity are:

1. Strategic consideration — potential business development/ opportunity review;
2. Financial, legal and operational analyses;
3. Option prioritization, selection and planning; and
4. Option implementation.

This four-step process (illustrated in Figure 3.1) provides a systematic approach to assessing potential revenue diversification and enhancement strategies, including new services, internal/external group programs and joint ventures.

Figure 3.1

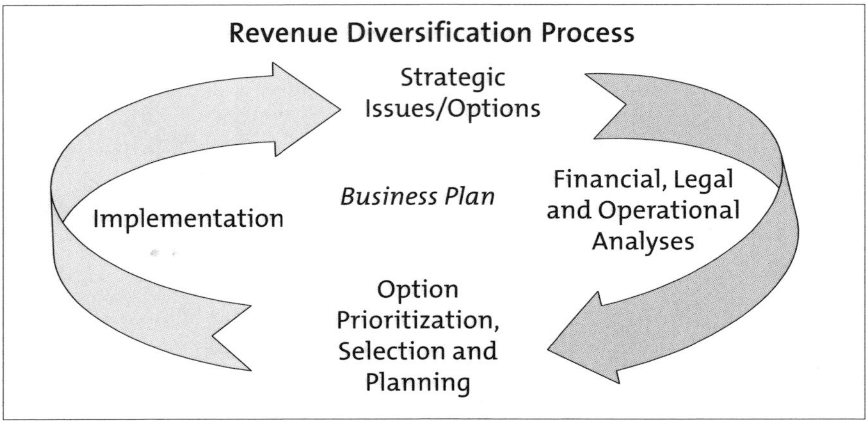

Revenue Diversification Process

Strategic Issues/Options

Implementation

Business Plan

Financial, Legal and Operational Analyses

Option Prioritization, Selection and Planning

An explanation of each phase in the process follows.

Strategic Issues/Options—potential business development/opportunity review

As a medical practice begins to consider how to enhance revenues and profits, its physician and administrative leadership will likely find that there are as many opinions or ideas as there are voices within the practice. The ultimate success of any revenue diversification strategy will depend on many factors, including selecting the right strategy and the level of physician and other buy-in for the chosen model. To promote and encourage physician commitment to a revenue-enhancing strategy, the practice leaders should examine various options openly and honestly. Ultimately the group's ownership must set the group's direction, clarify initiatives and formalize accountability.

A formal business development/opportunity assessment planning session that focuses on potential business initiatives encourages open discussion of potential revenue-enhancing initiatives. The session identifies the range of potential options and provides a means of coalescing the various opinions within the group into an acceptable scheme.

A strategic business development/opportunity assessment process should begin with a "laundry list" of potential revenue opportunities.

Items on the list include those that the group can or should consider, each of which must be viewed by at least one individual as a potential opportunity for additional revenues deemed worthy of further consideration. Create the list by asking one simple question: What types of services or revenue opportunities that are consistent with the organization's core business activities and service lines could be delivered that are not being delivered today? This question relates to the specific opportunities that may be available to the practice.

Today medical groups are pursuing many different revenue opportunities, including:

- Services that have historically been furnished by hospitals and hospital facilities, including diagnostic services (e.g., MRI, CT scan), cardiac catherization services and nuclear medicine.

- Freestanding diagnostic imaging centers.

- In-office and independent clinical laboratories.

- Investments in ambulatory surgery centers (ASCs).

- Emerging treatment methods, procedures, products and services that are consistent with provider specialties and clinically indicated (e.g., bariatric surgery, cosmetic (Botox) services, vein clinics).

- Alternative and complementary treatment therapies and modalities (e.g., acupuncture, psychological services).

In most instances, the medical group's core cluster of clinical services will serve as the foundation for the new revenue opportunity, but the diversification strategy will commonly focus on capturing an additional portion of the reimbursement dollar.

In some cases, however, the revenue opportunity may appear as part of a broader business plan directed at practice growth.

Draw initial conclusions as to the plausibility of each revenue enhancement initiative on the laundry list.

Get a "gut check" first. Are other groups successfully providing such services? Does your group have the resources or expertise required to implement the new services? Does it make sense to offer such services in light of the fundamental obligations of medical business outlined previously (i.e., clinically appropriate services furnished by competent providers in a legally compliant manner)? These questions will help you assess plausibility as well as rule out inappropriate initiatives.

Assess the internal strengths and weaknesses of the group as they relate to service delivery and support of each initiative.

What advantages does the group possess in terms of clinical expertise, managerial effectiveness and market position? Are any of those qualities deficient to the extent they may limit the success of an initiative?

Attempt to reach consensus on the most desirable initiative(s).

Rarely is there one clear revenue opportunity — a right or wrong way. The assessment process will require judgments about an uncertain future. And because the medical practice's providers may have diverse perspectives and member interests — which may all be legitimate — it is unlikely that the group members will reach unanimity on one preferred initiative. Nevertheless, the group will need to select plausible alternatives by prioritizing from the laundry list those initiatives that the group considers to have greatest potential short- and long-term benefit.

Factors to consider in determining the plausibility of each opportunity:

- External (those that the group cannot control):

  - Third-party payer reimbursement trends, including increases or decreases in third-party reimbursement models involving managed care, and increased willingness of patients to self-pay.

  - Population demographics of the practice's market area (i.e., youthful population, aging population).

  - Practice service-area economic conditions and stability.

  - Federal and state regulations and opportunities.

  - Current and potential competition for particular types of services.

- Internal (those that the group can control):

  - Current quality of care and patient services.

  - Operational conditions and efficiency.

  - Access and willingness to devote to capital to the venture.

  - Management expertise.

One effective way to conduct the business development/ opportunity assessment is through a retreat in which group owners, senior management and, sometimes, other participants clarify the practice's mission and goals as they relate to revenue enhancement and profit opportunities. A trained facilitator may help identify issues and/or concerns that may not be apparent to the group or may need clarification. A facilitator can push the participants to identify patterns, issues, necessary actions and implications of issue identification while maintaining the discussion and promoting decision making.

The initial strategic business development/opportunity assessment format promotes group cohesion. Group leaders demonstrate a willingness to consider all plausible revenue enhancement alternatives while setting a direction and action plan. The assessment format is not, however, designed to assess each potential alternative on financial, legal or other grounds. Rather, it identifies what the group considers its most plausible revenue enhancement opportunities. The process is designed to eliminate the "shotgun" approach to revenue diversification in favor of a structured and systematic design that fosters group cohesion and establishes a framework from which the financial assessment, legal analysis and prioritization of each conceptual initiative can begin.

The initial phase in the revenue diversification process consolidates the ideas that permeate the practice. It allows group members to discuss all plausible ideas, but, most importantly, it sets the direction for the group as it relates to revenue enhancement and/or diversification.

Using the SWOT Technique — Strengths, Weaknesses, Opportunities, Threats

A SWOT analysis provides a structured assessment of the strengths, weaknesses, opportunities and threats facing the medical group and its current activities.

A SWOT analysis helps clarify issues by juxtaposing two fundamental dimensions: good (strengths and opportunities) and bad (weaknesses and threats), or present (strengths and weaknesses) and future (opportunities and threats).

The SWOT process begins by framing the big picture. Answering these questions will help:

- What major revenue enhancement opportunities does the group have?

- What major external threats does the group face in relation to the opportunities identified?

- What are the major internal strengths within the group that would support each potential initiative?

- What are the group's weaknesses that would negate or marginalize each initiative, and that would therefore need to be overcome?

Financial, Legal and Operational Analysis

The strategic business development/opportunity assessment review phase described above establishes a set of specific initiatives that, through consensus building, are plausible and potentially acceptable for the medical practice. The group administrator will be a key participant during the strategic assessment process, generally responsible for assessing each initiative in a structured manner, considering financial, legal and operational issues.

Because legal issues are outlined in Chapter 4, our present focus will be on financial and operational considerations. A medical group should consider only those services that it can furnish without violating legal requirements and in a manner consistent with a practice's compliance culture and level of risk tolerance.

Each proposed initiative should be subjected to a standard financial evaluation method. Financial analysis projects the revenues likely to accrue from the development and implementation of a new revenue opportunity, guides the group in avoiding adverse effects from the wrong decision and helps it anticipate financial performance under alternative scenarios. The financial/analytical assessment required is straightforward and uncomplicated.

Factors for Financial Assessment:

- Demand for services

- Payer assessment and reimbursement per service

- Estimated revenues

- Projected expenses and cost per service

- Impact on practice operations

- Pro forma development using these factors.

Assessing Demand. The demand for each proposed revenue opportunity or ancillary service initiative is arguably the most important evaluation variable. It requires an objective assessment of likely volume or demand for a given product or service. Each of the evaluation variables that follow will be based on the expected demand. For example, an orthopedic practice considering the addition of extremity MRI services would likely weigh the following factors to establish potential demand for the services:

- Referrals out of the practice for MRI services for at least three months to address normal practice patterns and fluctuations;

- Out-referrals by payer mix to determine projected revenue by third-party payer-type, as well as to identify potential barriers created by existing third-party payer arrangements (i.e., those in which the group's furnishing of additional services would be viewed as out-of-network services or not paid for by existing payers);

- Patient demographics in the practice's primary and secondary markets as a means to assess the potential increased or decreased use of extremity MRI services in the future; and
- Patient preferences for a new service line or an alternative to existing service providers in the community.

Payer Assessment. Critical to the assessment process is a determination of how the group's payers will reimburse the practice for the proposed service. The group must review each payer contract and contact each payer to address issues related to the proposed revenue opportunity not clear in the contract.

Questions to Ask of Payers:

- Will the services and procedures associated with the proposed revenue opportunity constitute covered services under the contract?

- What is the reimbursement per applicable CPT code?

- Are there provisions in the third-party payer contract that allow the payer to designate where the proposed services are provided — either today or in the future?

- Are there annual maximum service levels?

- What CPT codes should be used for the services and what are the appropriate modifiers, if applicable?

- Will the payer actually pay for the service?

Ideally, the group would receive a letter from each payer stipulating answers.

The payer assessment of the revenue opportunity will provide critical information including the plans financial strengths and weaknesses. More often than not, the payer assessment provides a greater understanding that not every payer will cover the proposed services, and a greater appreciation of the potential barriers to payment under each contractual arrangement.

Estimating Revenue. Once the group has formalized the expected service demand and assessed third-party payer reimbursement, it can estimate service revenue. The revenue estimation process collects information to understand the potential financial implications of any particular revenue opportunity, and assists a practice in developing a fuller understanding of the potential financial implications under various scenarios.

Tables 3.1 through 3.4 illustrate one potential approach a group can use to project revenue based on a detailed review of estimated demand, reimbursement levels by third-party payers and related variables. Recognize that other, less sophisticated and data-driven approaches are also available as described below.

Because Medicare is the dominant payer for many practices and because many third-party payers base their reimbursement levels on percentages of Medicare, payment levels under the Medicare program provide a good starting point for the revenue projection process. Table 3.1 shows an assessment of global reimbursement under Medicare for MRI services.

Table 3.1. CPT and Medicare Reimbursement Levels
Select MRI Procedures

CPT		Non-Facility Total RVU	Payment Per Procedure
73718	MRI lower extremity w/o dye	12.67	$ 464.93
73719	MRI lower extremity w/ dye	15.20	557.66
73720	MRI lower extremity w/o & w/ dye	27.29	1,001.37
73721	MRI joint of lower extremity w/o dye	12.67	464.93
73722	MRI joint of lower extremity w/ dye	15.20	557.66
73723	MRI joint lower extremity w/o & w/ dye	27.29	1,001.37

Table 3.2 on the following page combines information collected in the demand and the payer assessment activities. In this example, the practice's demand assessment process revealed that during the prior 12-month period, the practice referred 399 MRI procedures in the select CPT code categories. Some practices have highly sophisticated information systems that allow them to determine the demand by service (i.e., CPT code) and by third-party payer (including subcategories of commercial payers). Many others, however, will only know aggregate estimates of procedure volumes. Even here, however, practices can make rough estimates based on volume by payer category by applying the overall payer mix to the volume estimates and assumptions. The result is an estimate of procedures by third-party payer category as illustrated in Table 3.2.

Table 3.2. Estimated procedures by Payer
Payer Mix Analysis – Volume

	Medicare	Medicaid	Commercial	Worker's Comp	Other	Total
% of Total Payers	25%	4%	54%	13%	4%	100%
CPT						
73718	31	5	66	16	5	123
73719	19	3	40	10	3	75
73720	1	0	3	1	0	5
73721	27	4	58	14	4	107
73722	21	3	44	11	3	82
73723	2	0	4	1	0	7
Totals	101	15	215	53	15	399

Table 3.3 continues the revenue build-up by combining estimated procedure volumes with reimbursement levels by third-party payer. This also reflects the fact that many payers base their reimbursement levels on percentages of Medicare allowable charges. Revenues provided in Table 3.3 are developed by multiplying the estimated reimbursement for each payer class (obtained through the payer assessment process) by the estimated volume of procedures for that payer class.

The degree of specificity represented in Tables 3.1 to 3.3 will not be available to every practice. While detailed analysis of this nature may help provide the fullest understanding of the potential implications of a particular revenue diversification strategy, groups can and will need to rely on less-sophisticated methods that require fewer estimates.

Alternative methods that involve less data but build on the same basic analytical principles include the use of average

	Medicare	Medicaid	Commercial	Worker's Comp	Other
Table 3.3. Estimated Reimbursement by Volume and Payer Class Payer Mix Analysis – Reimbursement by Payer Class by Estimated Demand/Volume					
Reimbursement as % of Medicare	100%	75%	135%	105%	100%
CPT					
73718	$14,180	$1,702	$41,350	$7,742	$2,269
73719	10,317	1,238	30,083	5,633	1,651
73720	1,252	150	3,650	683	200
73721	12,437	1,492	36,266	6,790	1,990
73722	11,432	1,372	33,336	6,242	1,829
73723	2,003	240	5,840	1,094	320
Totals	$51,621	$6,194	$150,525	$28,184	$8,259
			Grand Total		**$244,783**

reimbursement by CPT code coupled with estimates of total volume by CPT. Some practices will base their "first cut" financial analysis on Medicare rates, even though they fully expect that reimbursement levels — and therefore revenues — will be greater than Medicare's for a portion of their patient base. They take the view that if the revenue opportunity works with Medicare alone, it will most likely succeed when private-pay patients are included.

Assessing the Costs. The primary cost assessment should consider a number of key variables:

- Cost to acquire the technology, skills, etc., required for the new service, including costs to train physicians to learn a new service, purchase/lease of the equipment required for a new service, etc. (e.g., capital cost, interest, depreciation);
- Facility expense (required remodeling, rent, utilities, etc.);
- Staff cost (new staff, training, certification);
- Supplies (initial inventory and ongoing logistical support); and

- Maintenance agreement and/or expected annual repair expense.

These criteria may seem obvious, but oftentimes a practice omits important components of a cost analysis: opportunity cost and a determination of the cost per service (if applicable).

Don't Ignore Opportunity Costs

Opportunity costs refer to lost potential revenue. Using extremity MRI services as an example, if adding MRI service requires the conversion of two or more exam rooms, the lost revenue to the practice as a result of not having two exam rooms is an opportunity cost. The practice must weigh this opportunity cost against the projected revenue from extremity MRI services.

Even services that do not involve facility modifications or new equipment may involve opportunity costs. A general surgical practice might develop a specialization in bariatric surgery to alleviate severe obesity. The local hospital may assume the cost of capital and equipment for the surgical procedures, but the practice and one or more of its physicians will still have to pay for training to perform the new service or procedure. The lost revenues associated with the training period, salary support that the practice must provide during the training period and other expenses may also be appropriately viewed as opportunity costs associated with the practice's pursuit of the revenue opportunity.

Cost Per Service. Many groups determine the cost per service delivery. Use a relative value unit (RVU) cost system to provide a simple basis for cost allocation. RVUs measure the resources necessary to perform a procedure or deliver a unit of service and are used extensively to develop fees. There are several sources for obtaining specific formulas to develop RVU costing systems, Medicare's Resource-Based Relative Value Scale (RBRVS) being the most commonly used.

One often-used RVU approach is to aggregate all costs (i.e., labor, supplies, equipment, space) and determine the average cost per RVU for the practice as a whole by dividing total allocated costs by total RVUs for the number of procedures performed. For example, if the total nonphysician operating costs (excluding physician compensation and benefits) for an eight-physician orthopedic practice equals $2,296,312, and during the time period those costs were incurred the practice generated 114,608 total RVUs, the total cost per RVU would equal $20.03—total nonphysician operating cost divided by the total number of RVUs. This estimated cost per RVU would then be applied to the volume assumptions referenced above to estimate costs per service or procedure, as illustrated in Table 3.4.

Table 3.4. Estimated Cost per Procedure Based on RVUs			
Cost Analysis by CPT			
CPT	Non-Facility Total RVU	Cost Per Total RVU	Payment Per Procedure
73718	12.67	$20.04	$253.91
73719	15.20	20.04	304.61
73720	27.29	20.04	546.89
73721	12.67	20.04	253.91
73722	15.20	20.04	304.61
73723	27.29	20.04	546.89

Applying aggregate costs to all RVUs as illustrated above is one means of determining the approximate cost per service. However, more precise cost methodologies incorporate cost centers, direct/indirect cost determination and a specific allocation process, as suggested in the preceding chapter. For the purpose of a feasibility assessment, the total RVU methodology illustrated above is generally acceptable. The cost data—both in the aggregate and on a per unit of service basis—can be used in conjunction with demand, payer assessment, revenue and other data to construct financial pro forma—or forecasted financial statement—to assess the feasibility of a proposed revenue opportunity.

Impact on Practice Operations. After a practice has figured anticipated demand, direct costs, opportunity costs and projected revenue, it must also assess what the inclusion of the new service or initiative will have on the practice's overall operations. Each proposed revenue-enhancing initiative should be assessed in relation to ongoing group management, patient registration, claims processing, accounts receivable management, utilization review/quality assurance and required indirect support staff. Use the same evaluation criteria on all proposed initiatives.

Pro Forma Development. Once the evaluation criteria have been completed, the group should develop a pro forma that compares the projected revenues and costs over a specific period of time. A pro forma projects the future financial position for each plausible initiative, illustrating expected changes in cash flow over a specific period of time.

Table 3.5 presents a basic pro forma built from the combination of procedure codes and estimated demand, payer mix and cost per unit of service.

Table 3.5. Pro Forma
Pro forma estimated revenues and cost by CPT

CPT	Estimated Revenues (Volume by Payer x Reimbursement)	Estimated Cost (Volume x Cost per Service)
73718	$67,243	$30,969
73719	48,922	22,531
73720	5,936	2,734
73721	58,975	27,161
73722	54,211	24,967
73723	9,497	4,374
Opportunity Cost (Space, etc.)		60,000
Total	$244,784	$172,736
Estimated Profit (Loss)		**$72,048**

Appendix A presents a more detailed pro forma income statement. Please note that the format illustrated is designed only for the process of comparing and contrasting proposed initiatives, revenues and costs, and is not presented as a comprehensive future statement of a group's financial viability.

In addition to the basic pro forma of revenues, costs and estimated profits or losses from the revenue opportunity, a practice should also undertake a basic sensitivity analysis to more fully assess the assumptions and potential implications of alternative scenarios. Sensitivity analysis is little more than a process of applying alternative assumptions to the financial model used in the initial analysis.

For example, Table 3.6 below applies a sensitivity analysis to the financial projections illustrated in Tables 3.1 to 3.5 but slightly modifies the modeling assumptions. The conservative scenario posits that the MRI volume used in the basic analysis is overly aggressive, and instead assumes that only 60 % of the forecasted demand will exist. This type of assessment is critically important, as many practices will project overly optimistic levels of service volume or confront unexpected restrictions from third-party payers that will decrease service levels. Likewise, Table 3.6 presents potential scenarios of true growth in medically appropriate service volume. All assumptions use the same fixed cost structure without any change based on service volume, therefore imposing an additional conservative measure on the analysis.

Table 3.6. Sensitivity Analysis to Assess Different Assumptions and Scenarios			
	Conservative	Moderate	Growth
% of Current Volume	60%	100%	120%
CPT			
73718	$40,346	$67,243	$80,691
73719	$29,353	$48,922	$58,706
73720	$3,561	$5,936	$7,123
73721	$35,385	$58,975	$70,770
73722	$32,526	$54,211	$65,053
73723	$5,698	$9,497	$11,396
Estimated Total Revenue	$146,869	$244,784	$293,739
Estimated Cost	$112,736	$112,736	$112,736
Opportunity Cost	$60,000	$60,000	$60,000
Estimated Profit (Loss)	-$25,867	$72,048	$121,003

When assessing new revenue sources and/or services, a pro forma for three years is generally acceptable, given the changes in health care today.

Option Prioritization, Selection and Planning

Through the first two phases of the revenue diversification process the medical group has identified the plausible strategic initiatives designed to enhance its revenues. The initiatives are consistent with, conform to and support the group's mission and values. The group has also assessed the financial, legal and operational implications of each proposed initiative.

The third phase of the revenue diversification process involves the formal prioritization of the initiatives considered, coupled with the selection and planning of strategies incorporated as part of the group's overall business plan.

The group may also want to assess the impact of not implementing the revenue-enhancing initiatives being assessed.

A medical group generally formalizes the selection and prioritization phase by reconvening the individuals who participated in the business development/opportunity analysis session or a subset of those participants (i.e., board of directors or planning committee). They review, prioritize and ultimately select the initiative(s) for implementation. They should consider the findings of each of the previously discussed assessment criteria, i.e., demonstrated demand, legal issue consideration, projected revenues and costs, impact on operations and applicable subjective analyses. By reviewing the full set of data, the individuals participating in the selection process will identify the initiative(s) deemed appropriate for development and

> ## Don't forget the softer issues
>
> In addition to quantitative analysis, some initiatives may call for a group to consider more subjective factors. Subjective selection criteria may include the political acceptability of each initiative and the impact each initiative may have on:
>
> - Referral patterns;
>
> - Medical community cohesion;
>
> - Hospital relationship(s);
>
> - Patient perceptions of the group, its perceived quality of service and other factors; and
>
> - The community in general.

implementation, and gain a fuller understanding of the strengths, weaknesses, assumptions etc., associated with the proposed revenue opportunity and essential to the venture's prospects for success.

Implementation and Incorporation as Part of Overall Business Plan

Once the medical group has completed the selection and prioritization process, with the strategic initiatives identified and committed to, it needs to develop an operations/business plan to formalize tasks and operations and identify resources to support the established initiatives — including those specifically directed at the selected revenue-generating initiatives.

The business plan serves as a road map that details the starting point, direction and destination of group operations over a specific period. The plan need only address operational issues and events designed to support the adopted strategic initiatives. Historical trends or forecasting or evaluating environmental issues occurred in the business development/opportunity session or financial analysis phases.

The Making of the Business Plan

Components and order of development:

- Background — provides an overview of the group's development and structure.

- Mission statement — declares the group's purpose and services and identifies primary and secondary market areas.

- Goals/objectives — when met will lead to achieving the group's mission. Objectives commonly compose administrative/management services, accounting/financial services and marketing/organizational growth.

- Tactical strategies — events and operations that the group will accomplish to support its goals and objectives. Each selected revenue enhancement initiative should be presented as separate tactical strategy, and each tactical strategy should address issues of purpose, implementation, resource allocation, responsible parties and evaluation. State at least the following for each strategy:

- ▪ Purpose — what is the objective of the strategic initiative?

- ▪ Implementation — what is going to be done? How is the strategy/initiative going to be implemented, operated, monitored and evaluated?

- ▪ Resources — what resources will be committed for implementation, operation and monitoring?

- ▪ Individuals responsible for implementation, operations, monitoring and evaluation.

- ▪ Evaluation criteria.

- ▪ Timeframe for implementation and evaluation.

- ● Financial strategy — an expanded supporting pro forma budget/financial statement with descriptions of revenue, expenses and capital expenditures designed to support the adopted strategic initiatives and ongoing operations.

Rules of thumb:

- ● Focus the plan on the process and action or tactical activities, as well as desired outcomes.

- ● Keep the plan clear, concise and without superficial narratives.

- ● Ensure the plan remains flexible to respond efficiently to inevitable environmental and organizational changes.

- ● Include financial strategies (projected incomes/cash flow, operating budget) to support the group's tactical strategies and ongoing operations.

Consider the following when developing your plan:

- View the plan as an investment in the group's future success — not just as a great deal of work.

- Develop the plan with the components and in the order of development outlined above to maintain a focus on the practice as a whole, while setting the stage for the new revenue-generating ventures.

- Make the plan as succinct as possible — generally no more than 20 to 30 pages.

- Focus on the intended reader (e.g., group members, outside investors). Address questions or issues important to the intended audience.

- Be realistic. Base any projections on the results — both positive and negative — of the analysis.

- Evaluate the business plan at least quarterly.

- Involve staff in the plan's development, execution, monitoring and evaluation.

Avoid:

- Excessive time frame. Because the business and regulatory environments change rapidly, a formal business plan should not exceed more than three years in its outlook.

- Lack of specificity. To avoid confusion among leaders and staff, clearly define measurable objectives and process planning.

- Infrequent reviews. Evaluate the business plan every quarter and modify it if necessary to address organizational and environmental changes.

- Separate plans for all enterprising ventures. Too often, separate plans conflict, lack coordination and consistency, or do not conform to or support the overall plan of the group. The solution: one group, one plan.

- Failure to fully use the business plan. Use the plan to monitor progress, communicate with stakeholders, potential partners and financial backers, and even as a recruiting tool for new physicians.

- Keeping the plan a secret. Use it as a working document available to all staff, regardless of position. Staff must understand where the practice is going and how they can help it get there.

Know the Basics

- Do not underestimate the operational, financial and legal requirements of revenue-diversification activities.

- Observe the fundamental obligation of medical business — i.e., medically appropriate care furnished by competent personnel in compliance with applicable laws.

- Ensure that your medical group leadership has a shared vision of the future, an ability to change with the environment and understanding that medical groups must function as businesses.

- Follow a formal approach to identifying, evaluating and implementing revenue-diversification options.

- Employ sound business techniques to analyze diversification options.

- Implement your diversification strategies with a formal business plan that will serve as a road map to communicate goals, financial objectives and operational tactics.

CASE STUDY: Ambulatory Surgical Center Development

Background

In the late 1990s three orthopedic surgery, neurosurgery and neurology practices comprising 18 physicians began exploring a practice merger. During the pre-merger feasibility assessment, the groups established three goals related to clinical service delivery and revenue-enhancing ventures.

Revenue Diversification Goals

1. Promote medical and surgical care to the community and regional population with "one-stop shopping" convenience and service;
2. Maintain and enhance the merged group's revenue streams and income level *in spite of* declining reimbursement; and
3. Reduce overhead on a per-physician basis by applying ancillary income to overhead.

Business Development/Opportunity Review

In support of these goals, and following a formal planning session, the merging group prioritized the following potential service lines for additional consideration:

- Ambulatory surgery center (ASC)
- Magnetic resonance imaging (MRI)
- Physical therapy (PT)
- Durable medical equipment
- Pain center services

The prioritized assessment initially focused on ASC, MRI and PT services. The ASC presented the most complex review due to three potential alternative business models and the various opportunities and costs associated with each.

The three alternative models were: a same-day ASC joint venture with an integrated delivery system, participation in an existing ASC, or investment in an existing surgical center (Acme Surgical Center) that was licensed as a surgical hospital. These three models varied along a number of lines:

1. Ability to perform surgical procedures either on a same-day or overnight stay basis;
2. Reimbursement for various cases depending on payer source and procedure type;
3. Projected case volumes based on potential usage scenarios of each alternative facility; and
4. Financial return due to ownership interest available with the particular model.

To structure the analysis and evaluation process, a planning group developed five scenarios to compare the alternatives. The scenarios recognized the different capabilities of the three alternatives with the surgical hospital capable of serving a broader complement of cases than the ASC options, due to its overnight stay capabilities. The scenarios also recognized that not every eligible case would be furnished in a particular location due to patient choice, payer restrictions and other factors. The alternatives fell into five scenarios:

Scenario 1 Potential Acme Surgery Center Option — 100% of all procedures are performed at surgical hospital.

Scenario 2   Potential Acme Surgery Center Option — 75% of all procedures are performed at surgical hospital.

Scenario 3   Potential Acme Surgery Center Option — 60% of all procedures are performed at surgical hospital.

Scenario 4   ASC only — 100% option. No overnight stay cases and 100% of ASC-type cases performed in an ASC.

Scenario 5   ASC only — 75% option. No overnight stay cases and 75% of ASC-type cases performed in an ASC.

Demand and Payer Assessments

To assess demand the groups assumed that their existing surgical case mixes would continue with any merged practice. A spreadsheet was developed to identify and combine the procedures provided by the three groups that would make up the merged group. The spreadsheet contained the following data:

- CPT codes
- Procedure descriptions
- Expected volumes over a 12 month period
- Percent of Medicare patients
- Number of Medicare patients
- Estimated Medicare reimbursement
- Percent of private and commercial payers
- Number of private and commercial payers
- Estimated private and commercial reimbursement
- Estimated total reimbursement

This provided the group with information on the pool of surgical cases that a surgical center alternative could potentially furnish. The planning committee further pared this listing to:

1. Eliminate certain procedures for which no facility fee reimbursement in an ASC or surgical hospital would be provided;

2. Eliminate procedures performed by group surgeons outside of the local community;
3. Attribute 15% of all cases to Medicare reimbursement based on merged group's estimated payer mix; and
4. Develop estimate of average net revenue per surgical procedure to include professional component and facility fee.

Estimating Revenues

Procedures were estimated based on information provided by the groups, resulting in the following revenue estimate for the Acme Surgical Center alternative (assuming 100% of cases are performed in the surgical hospital):

	Total estimated surgical procedures	2,475
x	Average net revenue per procedure	$2,326
=	**Estimated annual net revenue**	**$5,756,850**

Cost Estimates

The groups estimated general operating expenses to estimate overall contribution margins, using the following assumptions:

- Professional staff salaries were based on an average salary of $43,000 and aggregate staff time of 10 hours per case.
- Fringe benefits were estimated at 25% of cash compensation.
- Medical supplies were estimated at $224.64 per case.
- General direct expenses were estimated at $48.63 per case.
- Annual occupancy expense (including debt service, taxes, and associated operating expenses estimated at $240,000).
- Equipment expense was based on the potential need for two to four operating rooms and associated recovery and support space, depending on the volumes associated with

each scenario. Financing was assumed at 80% of anticipated expenses and 8.75% interest for seven years.

- No provision was made for cost of surgical instruments.
- The current number of physicians was assumed with no provision for group growth.

Pro Forma Development

The revenue and cost assumptions outlined above were incorporated into financial pro forma designed to estimate the five alternative scenarios and the potential contribution of each model alternative. To provide for a conservative assessment, costs were maintained at a constant level (assuming costs for 100% usage) under all scenarios.

The following table presents an example of the pro forma based on Scenario No. 2— Acme Surgery Center option assuming 75% of all potential procedures are performed in the center.

Pro Forma—Scenario No. 2 Contribution Analysis	
	Total
Estimated procedures	1,857
Average net revenue per procedure	$2,326
Estimated annual net revenues*	**$4,319,382**
Estimated annual operating expenses:	
Salaries	$1,412,431
Fringe benefits (25%)	$353,108
Medical supplies	$555,984
General direct expenses	$120,359
Equipment expense (4 rooms)	$192,733
Annual occupancy expense (including debt service, taxes & operating expenses)	$240,000
Total estimated operating expenses	**$2,874,614**
Estimated contribution margin (including professional service income)	$1,444,768
Estimated professional service income	$(871,995)
Estimated contribution margin net of professional service income	$572,773

Estimated annual net revenues includes approximately $871,995 in professional fee net revenue attributed to group physicians who used the Acme Surgery Center.

Decision

Following the various analyses, the group purchased a 51% ownership in the Acme Surgery Center. The primary reasons for this decision:

- Higher estimated revenues and contribution margin
- Broader scope of procedures
- Ability to service more complex cases and cases with higher reimbursement levels
- No certificate of need (CON) requirement
- Cases can begin immediately
- Mostly physician-owned
- Located in the growing area of the new group's service area

Realized Benefits of the Surgical Center Investment:

1. Highly satisfactory annual revenue stream from surgical center operations;
2. Enhanced ability to recruit neuromuscular specialty physicians; and
3. Help to enforce "one-stop shopping" for the region's population in need of neuromuscular services.

CASE STUDY: Shared Cardiology Diagnostic Center

Background

A medical office building in a growing suburb of a large urban area houses two small medical practices specializing in general internal medicine and noninvasive cardiology. A large cardiology group operates a clinical practice outreach site in the same building. The three groups and providers have historic relationships as friendly competitors coupled with referral and patient care relationships, as physicians in the smaller practices have historically referred patients to the larger group for invasive and interventional cardiology services.

Each of the smaller practices had independently examined the possible development of in-house echocardiography, nuclear medicine and similar cardiac diagnostic capabilities. Each practice had historically used hospital-based diagnostic resources to furnish the diagnostic services. The two small practices had each conducted independent analyses and concluded that neither group had sufficient patient volume to justify the space, equipment, personnel and other costs that would be associated with developing an in-house cardiac diagnostic center. However, due to regulatory changes associated with the federal physician self-referral or Stark law, which allow for certain shared facility arrangements, the two small groups elected to approach the larger cardiology group about developing a shared facility.

Pro Forma Development and Sensitivity Analysis

The three practices performed financial analyses related to the venture using alternative assumptions related to the historic service volumes. They used three volume assumptions: moderate (same as historic volume), conservative (75% of historic volume), and growth (125% of historic volume) scenarios. They assumed that expenses remained constant under the conservative and moderate scenarios, while increasing certain expense categories under the growth scenario.

Pro forma projections for nuclear medicine procedures are illustrated in the following table.

Pro Forma – Nuclear Medicine			
	Conservative	Moderate	Growth
Revenue: Nuclear			
X patients (100)	$54,375	$72,500	$90,625
Y Patients (115)	$62,531	$83,375	$104,219
Z patients (720)	$391,500	$522,000	$652,500
Supply Income (assume wash)	$128,000	$128,000	$160,000
Total nuclear revenue	$636,406	$805,875	$1,007,344
Expense: Nuclear			
Human resource expense	$116,000	$116,000	$156,000
Equipment lease expense	$120,000	$120,000	$120,000
Rental expense	$14,700	$14,700	$14,700
Service contract	$6,000	$6,000	$6,000
Depreciation	$8,400	$8,400	$8,400
Pharmacy	$128,000	$128,000	$160,000
Other	$40,000	$40,000	$40,000
Total nuclear expense	$433,100	$433,100	$505,100
Profit contribution nuclear	$203,306	$372,775	$502,244

Legal Compliance

In the current regulatory environment some, but not all of the services furnished through the shared facility would be paid for by Medicare and subject to the Stark law's self-referral prohibitions, including echocardiography procedures. Nuclear medicine procedures are not presently defined as designated health services and therefore are not subject to the Stark law.

Despite the above, the Phase I final rule to the Stark law allows for the use of shared facilities in furnishing designated health services, provided that the physicians and medical groups sharing the facility furnish and bill for all services in compliance with the Stark law's in-office ancillary services exception. And although at the time of the venture, nuclear medicine services were not subject to the Stark law's self-referral prohibitions, the practices and providers approached the venture with the working assumption that such services could, at some point, become subject to the Stark law restrictions. The operational practices for the shared facility structure and the three medical groups' internal operations (e.g., scheduling, physician supervision) were therefore crafted to promote compliance with these requirements.

In addition to Stark law compliance, the financial arrangements between the practices and providers are structured to promote compliance with the antikickback statute by allocating the costs and expenses of the shared facility based on a fair market value assessment. Other contractual and related safeguards are instituted to promote compliance.

CASE STUDY: MRI

Background

An eight-physician orthopedic group practice providing services in the subspecialties of sports medicine, total joint replacement, spine, foot and ankle, pediatrics, shoulder, and elbow and hand considered providing MRI services.

Financial/Legal and Operational Assessment Phase

The group requested CPT code and volume data for extremity MRI procedures that were referred to local MRI providers (free-standing open MRI and hospital) to determine the number of extremity MRIs historically ordered by group physicians. The practice reviewed its private payer contracts and contacted the local payers to determine estimated reimbursement levels for extremity MRI services. It also contacted another private practice in a different market area of the state that furnished extremity MRI services to confirm that payer reimbursement was not an issue.

The group determined the operational requirements associated with the extremity MRI. Group leaders determined that the practice had adequate space for an extremity MRI within the existing physical plant. They identified the additional operational requirements required, including lead-lined walls, a special door to the MRI room, a printer for MRI scans, extremity MRI equipment and training of physicians and staff. It determined that a new heating, ventilation and air-conditioning (HVAC) system would be required for the MRI room, along with new flooring and other fixtures. The group identified an extremity MRI that was available under a five-year lease and maintenance agreement.

As part of the feasibility assessment process the group also obtained legal guidance on the ability to operate an in-house MRI. The group would need to meet these requirements regarding the distribution of MRI income in light of the Stark law, and reimbursement and related requirements associated with radiology over-reads of the MRI scans. The practice and its physicians committed to operating any MRI in compliance with applicable laws.

The group estimated expenses associated with the MRI to include salaries, equipment lease, space, supplies, radiologists' reading fees, etc. It coupled these with revenue projections based on historic demand and reimbursement levels from third-party payers. The revenue and expense data allowed the group to determine that an average of 1.5 scans per day would be required for the new venture to break even.

As part of the assessment project the group also performed a cash flow projection to estimate the potential start-up costs and expenses associated with the new venture. It conducted a sensitivity analysis to assess likely financial implications if demand and revenue projections were not met, excerpts of which are provided in the table shown on the following page:

Cash Flow Analysis

| | | Month | | | | | | | | | |
	Pre-Open	1	2	3	4	5	6	7	Etc.	12	Total
Revenues											
Capital contribution	$50,000										
Charges		$8,160	$9,600	$12,000	$14,400	$14,400	$14,400	$14,400	Etc.	$14,400	$159,360
Receipts		$-	$-	$-	19,344	23,400	26,520	28,080	Etc.	28,080	$237,744
Year-to-date		$-	$-	$-	19,344	42,744	69,264	97,344	Etc.	237,744	
Total receipts											$237,744
Expenses											
Development	$50,000										
Building		$3,200	$3,200	$ 3,200	$3,200	$3,200	$3,200	$3,200	Etc.	$3,200	
Equipment		8,333	$8,333	8,333	8,333	8,333	8,333	8,333	Etc.	8,333	
Staff		3,120	3,120	3,120	3,120	3,120	3,120	3,120	Etc.	3,120	
Supplies		417	417	417	417	417	417	417	Etc.	417	
Etc.		Etc.									
Total estimated cost	$50,000	$8,788	$8,788	$ 8,788	$8,788	$8,788	$8,788	$8,788	Etc.	$8,788	$155,456

Net Profit $82,288

Planning and Implementation

After determining the financial, legal and operational feasibility of the project, the group focused on planning and implementation. Leaders considered a variety of factors: staffing concerns (including technician training and services); alternative meeting space, as the MRI would be housed in a practice meeting room; scheduling and managing the facility redesign and build-out.

The group also weighed operational concerns including modifications in appointment scheduling, protocol development for chart flow including dictation and charge tickets. The group completed a contract with a local radiology group to provide over-reads and established a payment arrangement that was consistent with fair market value. The over-read process required that the group develop and implement a protocol for completion of all dictation, as well as a reconciliation process to eliminate any missing MRI dictation and reports.

Leaders developed a quarterly evaluation study. They also drew up an outcome study to ensure the group implemented all practices in accordance with agreed-upon protocols. The group also conducted an outcome study for future medical education.

Realized Benefits of In-house MRI Services

- Greater flexibility in patient schedules and convenience for extremity MRI services – especially for out-of-town patients;

- Enhanced efficiency in making timely diagnoses, therefore expediting medical care;

- Same or enhanced service quality through use of radiologist over-reads; and

- Additional revenues to support practice operations and incomes.

Legal/Structural Considerations and Alternatives

The revenue-diversification opportunities available to a particular practice will vary. The options available to a provider will depend in large part on the nature of the medical group and its resources.

Chapter 3 outlined the basic process to explore revenue diversification opportunities, and stressed that financial, operational and legal concerns are relevant to an appropriate analysis. The financial and operational analysis reviewed in Chapter 3 may, among other things, help a practice evaluate whether it can develop a proposed revenue opportunity independently, or whether it will need the involvement of other health care providers or third parties. Thus, the analysis of business-related issues will suggest structural options and alternatives, and those alternatives will, in turn, be influenced by the legal and regulatory environment.

Figure 4.1 on page 63 illustrates some of the structural models and options medical groups can use to pursue new revenue opportunities. While not an exhaustive summary of all potential alternatives, Figure 4.1 also shows the relationship among key variables of cost, complexity and business and legal risk. Some revenue opportunities can be pursued by a medical practice or even individual providers independently through the acquisition of additional skills or the lease or purchase of a new machine. Beyond these relatively small, incremental development activities, many groups will have a sufficient patient base and other advantages to pursue more elaborate ventures such as diagnostic clinics and surgical centers without the involvement of third parties.

In other cases, however, patient volume, capital, expertise or other needs will necessitate that the practice pursue revenue-diversification strategies through partnership arrangements. Such partnerships can range from shared facility arrangements to ventures involving the acquisition of specialized expertise, business management or support services from third-party organizations, to more traditional joint ventures in which the parties create an entirely new business enterprise and share the opportunity for profit and risk of loss.

Figure 4.1.

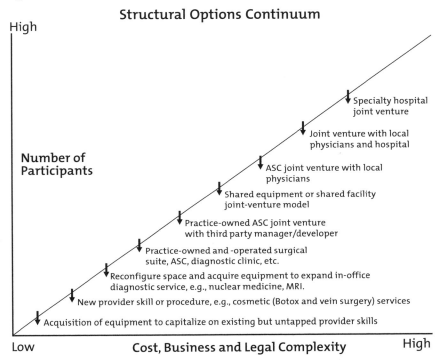

Regardless of the business strategy and revenue opportunity selected, each will come with varying degrees of legal complexity and risk. Figure 4.1 also illustrates the general rule that the demands of a project — whether measured in terms of cost, business complexity or legal compliance burdens — will generally diminish when only one provider or provider organization is involved, and when the revenue opportunity merely expands or builds on an existing service line, rather than a new line of business.

By illustration, a revenue opportunity or venture that involves a single physician learning a new procedure imposes fewer demands and is less complex than the development of an ambulatory surgical center that is wholly owned and operated by a single medical group. Similarly, the group-operated ASC will generally have less burden and complexity than a joint venture involving third parties, such as other physician groups, hospitals and others. Costs, managerial and legal complexity, and demands tend to increase as the sophistication and the number of "moving parts" required for the revenue opportunity increases.

A medical group must consider numerous legal and regulatory issues in connection with the development and implementation of a legally compliant revenue-diversification strategy. Some legal proscriptions will stand as potential barriers to the new venture, while others may actually create new opportunities. This chapter reviews some of the most important requirements and opportunities created by these laws and regulations, along with case study examples to illustrate structural options. Of course, each revenue-diversification strategy requires its own detailed, fact-specific analysis and guidance. Experience demonstrates that medical groups can develop legally compliant business models when the revenue opportunity involves multiple providers, complex business and service delivery models.

Key Legal Considerations

- Self-referral prohibitions

- Antikickback law

- Tax-exempt organization rules

- Federal reimbursement requirements

- Other state and federal laws and regulations

Self-Referral Prohibitions. The federal physician self-referral, or "Stark," law has commonly been viewed as the most significant barrier to revenue-diversification ideas. The law prohibits physicians from making referrals for certain "designated health services" (DHS) paid for by Medicare or Medicaid to entities with which the physician (or an immediate family member) has a financial relationship, *unless* an exception applies. DHS include clinical laboratory services, physical therapy services, diagnostic radiology services and inpatient and outpatient hospital services. The law prohibits both physician referrals and billing by entities that furnish DHS as a result of prohibited referrals.

Until recently, the Stark law created considerable uncertainty for health care business ventures due to its complexity, potentially harsh sanctions and the lack of final rules to clearly define the law's meaning. Phase I of the final rule implementing the Stark law became effective on Jan. 4, 2002, and provides much needed guidance related to some but not all of the Stark law's provisions. The still-forthcoming Phase II of the final rule will address additional Stark law provisions that may also help in revenue-diversification strategies. Importantly, the Stark law and the Phase I final rule have also clarified that certain revenue opportunities remain for physicians and medical groups *despite* the law's restrictions.

The Stark Law ...

- Prohibits physicians from making referrals for certain "designated health services" (DHS) paid for by Medicare or Medicaid, to entities with which the physician (or an immediate family member) has a financial relationship, *unless* an exception applies.

Some of the hidden opportunities existing at the time of publication include:

- Clarification that certain investments and services are not governed by the Stark law's self-referral prohibitions (e.g., nuclear medicine procedures, interests in ambulatory surgical centers and certain diagnostic services).

- Allowing medical groups and physicians to use "shared facilities" to furnish radiology, clinical laboratory and other DHS that are subject to the Stark law's proscriptions.

- Enabling medical practices to own and operate wholly owned laboratories, diagnostic imaging centers, physical and occupational therapy and other facilities — a structural alternative that can enable medical groups to furnish services to their own patients and to those referred to the facilities by other health care providers.

- The Stark law exception for "hospital ownership" that allows surgical, cardiology and other medical groups and their physicians to own and operate heart hospitals, surgical hospitals and other special hospital facilities.

- New opportunities for joint venture arrangements in rural communities that are created by the Stark law's rural provider exception.[1]

---

1. While these and other opportunities are currently available under the Stark law, the complex, changing nature of the health care legal and regulatory landscape must be considered in connection with any revenue-diversification strategy. By illustration, proposals in the Medicare reform legislation being debated by Congress in September 2003 would change the Stark law's "whole hospital" and rural provider exceptions. At press time these initiatives did not have the force of law. They illustrate, however, the potentially shifting landscape of regulatory compliance issues, suggesting that medical practices will be advised to: recognize that today's new venture may not last forever; anticipate and plan for exit strategies in connection with new venture development; and monitor the legal and regulatory landscape before, during and after developing a new ancillary service or other revenue diversification venture.

CASE STUDY: Wholly Owned Diagnostic Center

A medium-sized multispecialty medical group develops a wholly owned diagnostic center as an extension of the medical group's office-based practice. The center furnishes a host of services, including MRI, bone density X-ray, ultrasound procedures and echocardiography. Some but not all of the diagnostic services are DHS and subject to the Stark law's self-referral prohibitions. By relying on the Stark law's in-office ancillary services exception, the medical group can furnish and bill for diagnostic services payable by Medicare and Medicaid.

The only other available provider of many of the diagnostic services in the community is the local hospital. Accordingly, the medical group elects to qualify the center as an independent diagnostic treatment facility (IDTF) for Medicare payment purposes. The IDTF can accept referrals from, and provide technical component services to patients referred by physicians outside of the medical group. The medical group's diagnostic facility and the IDTF function as a shared facility for Stark law compliance purposes.

CASE STUDY: Office-Based Clinical Lab/ Independent Clinical Laboratory

---

A large medical group in an urban area operates a CLIA-certified clinical laboratory as part of the group's normal office-based practice. The group also operates the lab as a separate independent clinical laboratory under the Medicare program. This enables the group to furnish clinical laboratory services to patients of physicians outside of the medical group. The group's office-based clinical laboratory and the independent clinical laboratory are operated in compliance with applicable CLIA requirements, and as shared facilities as allowed under the Phase I final rule to the Stark law. The group also pays close attention to compliance with applicable state laws (e.g., licensure, certification) in developing and operating the venture.

CASE STUDY: Shared DEXA-Scan Facility

Two medical practices specializing in orthopedics and rheumatology located in the same office building form a joint venture to develop DEXA-scan capability to perform bone density studies. The practices identify the CPT codes for the studies and determine that such services are now subject to the Stark self-referral prohibitions, although they recognize that the services might become subject to the Stark law in the future. They conclude that they should craft their business model and legal structure on the assumption that Stark compliance may ultimately be necessary. The practices select a separate limited-purpose joint venture (JV) company owned by both practices as an appropriate business model.

The practices use the JV company to purchase the DEXA-scan machine, employ the technicians required for the studies, and lease the space used for the DEXA-scan equipment and services. The JV company leases use of the facility—including space, equipment and personnel—to each of the practices on a block-of-time basis. The groups bill for the DEXA-scan services under each practice's respective billing number.

Because the two practices periodically refer patients to each other, they pay close attention to ensuring that underlying financial, contractual and other relationships are consistent with fair-market value and crafted to promote compliance with an applicable safe harbor under the antikickback law. The block-of-time arrangement is also crafted to promote compliance with other Medicare and related reimbursement requirements, including those related to diagnostic test supervision and purchased diagnostic tests.

Antikickback Law. The federal antikickback law prohibits the payment of any remuneration — essentially anything of value — in exchange for federal health-care program patient service opportunities. Antikickback law violations constitute a felony criminal offense, punishable by imprisonment of up to five years, fines up to $25,000, or both, and sanctions may be imposed on all parties to an illegal transaction. Unlike violations of the Stark law, which requires no improper intent to violate the law, antikickback violations hinge on the parties' underlying intent.

The antikickback statute is sufficiently broad that any number of transactions and relationships between health care providers and entities can have potential antikickback implications, including joint-venture arrangements involving medical groups, physicians and other health care providers. Because the law has been in effect for an extended time, a significant body of regulatory and other guidance from the Office of Inspector General (OIG), U.S. Department of Health and Human Services is available regarding the law's application to a variety of business transactions.

Antikickback Guidance

Resources that provide guidance relating to revenue-diversification transactions that will not be treated as violating the antikickback statute include:

- "Safe harbor" regulations dealing with investments in ASCs, space and equipment leases, and personal service and management contracts;

- Favorable advisory opinions approving business arrangements involving joint-venture facilities for the delivery of health care services;

- Legal counsel with expertise in health care regulatory and compliance matters; and

- Information from these and other sources that can inform the structure and operating format of a host of provider organizations — including specialty hospitals, ASCs and imaging centers — while minimizing compliance risk.

The guidance related to the antikickback law by no means eliminates all uncertainty related to joint-venture and other arrangements that may be part of any revenue-diversification strategy. Nevertheless, this guidance provides sufficient structure to the health care delivery environment to enable providers to create business structures that are both legally compliant and competitive in today's changing marketplace.

CASE STUDY: Joint-Venture Ambulatory Surgical Center

Three orthopedic group practices develop and operate a joint-venture ambulatory surgical center. Each medical group retains its own independent identity, but each forms a separate limited liability company (LLC) entity to own the group's respective interests in the ASC. This structure is preferred for its ability to provide greater transferability and flexibility with respect to the ASC ownership interests.

These investment interests are structured to comply with the requirements of applicable antikickback law safe harbors. As a result, investors in the joint-venture ASC perform a significant number of surgical procedures in the ASC, and derive a significant portion of their income from procedures that can be performed in the facility. The physicians who use the ASC view it and use the facility as an extension of their practice.

Physicians performing procedures in the ASC receive compensation for their professional services under Medicare Part B. The ASC receives compensation for the facility services under the ASC composite rate structure. ASC services are not governed by the Stark law's self-referral prohibitions because they are paid for under the ASC composite rate structure.

CASE STUDY: Joint-Venture Imaging Center – Rural Area

Physicians in a rural community develop a joint-venture imaging center (JV Imaging Center). The center provides MRI, CT and other imaging services to patients from the local area and surrounding communities. The physicians own interests in the JV imaging center as allowed under the Stark law exception for ownership and investment interests in rural providers. As a result, the investing physicians can own interests in, and make referrals to, the JV imaging center for diagnostic services without violating the Stark law.

The investment interests in the JV imaging center fail to meet an applicable safe harbor under the antikickback statute. Nevertheless, the parties structure the venture to promote compliance with the proscriptions of the statute itself. Safeguards are incorporated into the JV imaging center's business model, capital structure and other arrangements to minimize the possibility that its purpose is to induce or reward referrals. Those safeguards relate to the nature of investment opportunity (i.e., investor benefits, investor selection and retention criteria), the joint venture's financing and profits distribution methodology, and business justification.

Tax-Exempt Organization Issues. While many medical groups will elect to go it alone in developing a new venture, some will partner with their local hospitals. For many hospitals and their physician partners, the laws and rules governing the activities of tax-exempt organizations will serve as an additional layer of regulatory compliance.

Hospitals and other health care organizations that enjoy tax-exempt status pursuant to Internal Revenue Code Section 501(c)(3) must be organized and operated exclusively for charitable purposes. Violations of I.R.C. § 501(c)(3) may result in the loss of an organization's tax-exempt status. Revenue diversification arrangements involving a tax-exempt hospital in a joint venture or partnership format can create legal concerns for Section 501(c)(3) hospitals. The IRS will assess whether the exempt organization's participation in the venture furthers an exempt purpose, and whether the arrangement permits the exempt body to act exclusively in furtherance of recognized exempt purposes. These and related requirements would have implications for the structure of any joint-venture arrangement, including the arrangement's governance, financing and other business terms. A practice seeking a revenue-diversification venture that involves a tax-exempt partner must consider and scale these hurdles — but experience demonstrates that they are by no means insurmountable.

CASE STUDY: Joint-Venture Specialty Hospital

A general acute care hospital and members of its medical staff develop a joint-venture specialty hospital to provide cardiovascular services. The new facility furnishes hospital services to the specialty hospital's inpatients, and is paid for those services under Medicare Part A. The specialty hospital is organized as a for-profit limited liability company (LLC) that provides pass-through partnership tax treatment to the specialty hospital's owners.

Because of the hospital's status as a Section 501(c)(3) tax exempt organization, leaders create governance and control structures to promote the hospital's charitable mission while reasonably promoting the economic and other interests of the specialty hospital's physician investors. The hospital is considering similar joint-venture arrangements with members of the medical staff specializing in orthopedic surgery, neurosurgery and certain other surgical specialties.

Services paid for as inpatient and outpatient hospital services under Medicare are defined as DHS under the Stark law, yet physicians own investment interests in the specialty hospital in reliance on the Stark law's exception for hospital ownership. Professional services of physicians who perform services in a specialty hospital do not constitute DHS, so escape the Stark law's self-referral prohibitions. Other compensation arrangements involving the specialty hospital and physicians (i.e., via medical director, lease and similar arrangements) are structured to comply with applicable Stark law exceptions, including those governing personal service arrangements and rental of space or equipment.

The ownership interests in the surgical hospital do not conform with an investment interest's safe harbor under the antikickback law. Nevertheless, the interests and underlying business terms are structured to provide distributions of profits based on equity rather than usage to promote Stark and anti-kickback law compliance.

CASE STUDY: Other Potential Arrangements

Other potential revenue enhancement strategies include:

- In-office cardiac catherization laboratories;
- Wholly owned comprehensive outpatient rehabilitation facilities (CORFs);
- New service lines (e.g., bariatric surgery services); and
- Sleep clinics and laboratories.

Many of the services furnished through such facilities are not defined as designated health services under the Stark law, or the services are subject to specific exceptions or exclusions under the law. Other laws, including state self-referral and antikickback prohibitions, facility licensure and certificate of need may be relevant to the development of a legally compliant enterprise, depending on the jurisdiction. In many settings medical groups may provide these types of services as part of, or in conjunction with, their traditional service base.

Federal Reimbursement Requirements. A host of other federal regulations related to reimbursement may also present untapped opportunities for various revenue-diversification strategies:

- Medicare Part B provides coverage of facility fees for services furnished in *Medicare-certified ASCs.* Entities that obtain state licensure and meet certain other requirements as required for Medicare certification are paid a composite rate that covers the cost of supplies, nursing services and equipment furnished through the ASC.

- Regulatory provisions allowing for the operation of *independent diagnostic testing facilities* (IDTF) that can be operated in conjunction with medical group-owned and -operated imaging and other diagnostic capabilities.
- *Independent laboratories* that can be operated by medical groups and furnish services to patients referred to the laboratory by physicians outside of the group.
- *Other special-purpose providers/suppliers* and service capabilities under Medicare rules.

While various reimbursement requirements may present untapped opportunities for revenue-stream diversification, each will also be accompanied by service-specific rules imposing requirements that must be complied with, including those related to levels of supervision, location of service delivery, billing arrangements and others. Practices must comply with all such requirements for payment under the Medicare and other Federal Health Care Programs. For example, a practice must consider Medicare rules governing purchased diagnostic tests in developing a legally compliant shared-facility venture. It must address local medical review policies of Medicare carriers in connection with the planning, design and operation of the venture. Although these regulatory requirements require close attention to promote compliance, new opportunities also exist in these areas. For example, the intersection of the Stark law's supervision requirements in the group practice context, and the supervision requirements governing many diagnostic services present opportunities not available before publication of the Stark law final rule.

Other Laws and Regulations. Aside from the federal statues referenced above, a medical group must also check other federal and state laws and regulations for regulatory compliance purposes. These include state certificates of need and laws and rules relating to licensure of hospitals and other health care facilities that provide outpatient medical services. State laws that impose "mini Stark" and "mini antikickback" prohibitions should also be identified early in the planning and assessment process. Such provisions commonly impose requirements that may mirror or approximate the requirements of the federal law counterparts. Not every state has versions of these laws, but those that do tend to present wide variations, thus mandating close legal review.

Many of the same federal and state laws and rules that have historically served as deal-killers in the past continue to act as threshold compliance hurdles. This factor is particularly important if payment for services by Medicare and other public payment systems is an essential element of a viable business model. Increasingly, however, a practice's Medicare participation is no longer essential to the success of many revenue-diversification strategies, and the group will offer the revenue opportunity exclusively to commercial and self-pay patients.

The second phase of the revenue-diversification process includes an assessment of legal as well as financial and operational feasibility. Addressing legal issues early on—at least through an initial assessment—will enable practices to avoid impractical revenue-diversification strategies, while structuring the models to promote appropriate compliance from the venture's inception.

Range of Issues to Consider

While the range of specific issues a practice will need to consider will vary depending on the particular revenue-diversification strategy, the list of potential considerations will include the following:

Federal

1. Stark self-referral issues

2. Antikickback issues

3. Medicare reimbursement

   - Service coverage and reimbursement limitations

   - Supplier/provider reimbursement categories, e.g., IDTF, CORF, ASC — opportunities and associated requirements

   - Reassignment issues

   - Billing and supervision requirements

   - Diagnostic test supervision requirements

   - Purchased diagnostic test rules

   - Clinical Laboratory Improvement Act (CLIA) requirements

4. Tax-exempt organization (I.R.C. Section 501(c)(3)) concerns (with hospitals and other partners)

5. Other federal tax considerations

State

6. State "mini Stark" prohibitions

7. State antikickback and similar provisions

8. Licensure and certification requirements under State law, e.g., hospital, ASC, clinic or similar license requirements coupled with mandated emergency room or emergency treatment requirements

9. Certificate of need

10. Medical practice act, corporate practice of medicine and similar professional licensure issues

11. State fee-splitting prohibitions

12. State tax considerations (e.g., excise and franchise taxes)

13. Health and safety provisions associated with particular activities

14. Local land use, zoning, environmental and similar restrictions

Structural Considerations

15. Structural relationships for venture, e.g., within existing organization, joint venture model, contractual relationships, wholly owned subsidiary

16. Form of entity considerations, e.g., business or professional corporation, limited liability company, limited liability partnership

17. Method of financial return, e.g., compensation for services, return on investment or both

18. Federal and state laws related to information disclosure and sale of securities such as stocks, bonds and other investment vehicles through equity and debt.

19. Capitalization and equity considerations, e.g., ownership shares, capitalization requirements, capital contributions vs. loans

20. Governance and decision-making

   - Board/committee structure

   - Owner vs. board/manager decisions

   - Majority and supermajority requirements

21. Organizational documents, service and contractual relationships

The legal and regulatory environment governing health care is obviously burdensome and complex. Yet a medical practice can successfully navigate them in today's emerging regulatory environment. The challenge for all health care providers is to craft a successful business model that will also promote legal compliance.

Know the Basics

The spectrum of new business opportunities tends to follow a structural continuum of cost, complexity and risk/reward.

- Legal and regulatory considerations may inhibit or facilitate revenue-diversification strategies.

- Both federal and state laws will govern many medical business activities.

- Regulatory uncertainty necessitates thorough consideration of myriad, complex issues.

- Seek appropriate legal review in connection with any new revenue program.

Business Considerations and Development Strategy Checklist

Every strategy deserves its own independent analysis in business, financial and legal terms. Physicians, medical groups, hospitals and other providers considering revenue opportunities will be well served by considering the following basic questions before embarking on any revenue-diversification strategy.

❑ **What are the revenue opportunities?** Services that are generally consistent with an organization's core health care service line will typically constitute the available revenue opportunities. Beyond those core business and service capabilities, many groups will consider more diverse, innovative and potentially risky strategies. These are the products and services that will define the universe of potential revenue opportunities.

❑ **Who will pay for the services, and how much?** Having a great idea is one thing, but the new revenue opportunities must result in payment for services. Some business models will rely entirely on private-pay patients — thus reducing compliance burdens. Others will only be economically feasible with access to patients covered by Medicare, Medicaid and other public-sector reimbursement systems.

☐ **What are the venture's potential up- and down-sides?** Not every venture will succeed, and some will fail. As part of the assessment process consider estimates of revenues and expenses. Financial analyses of potential best- and worst-case scenarios will be central to an evaluation of revenue-diversification options.

☐ **What laws and rules will apply?** The federal Stark law is not the only law that relevant to a revenue-diversification strategy, but it's a good place to start when assessing feasibility. Some services will constitute designated health services and will be subject to the law's prohibitions. Moreover, practices can structure some viable business models without having to rely on Medicare or public-pay business. Understanding the applicable regulatory environment is an essential step in developing a viable business venture.

☐ **What will be required to make the new venture work?** Operational, logistical and other factors must be considered early on in the planning process, in addition to financial and legal aspects. Groups should also recognize more subjective (and political) factors.

☐ **Who will be involved?** Can the medical group pursue the diversification strategy alone or will it need third parties' involvement? Some new ventures will succeed only when hospitals, specialized management companies or other parties actively participate in the enterprise through joint venture or other partnering arrangements.

❑ **How does the new venture relate to the practice's broader activities and strategies?** Successful ventures tend to build upon a practice's core functions while being integrated into the practice's larger strategic vision. Does the new venture truly fit the practice's business model, or will it demand so much time and attention that it risks sinking the entire ship?

❑ **Do practice physicians truly understand and support what is involved?** Physician buy-in is *always* critical to the success of a new revenue opportunity. Do the physicians in the practice truly understand, support and recognize both the costs and potential benefits of the new opportunity? Do they view the venture as an essential part of the practice or consider it a pet project of one or two physicians, the administrator or others?

❑ **Are adequate resources being devoted to help ensure success?** Development of a new business line on a shoestring without appropriate allocation of resources will often serve as an impediment to business success. Resources include capital available to purchase and lease equipment, renovate facilities and support training, but also time freed up to support marketing and patience with the opportunity and other costs that accompany the new venture. Are such costs and resources considered as part of the grand strategy?

❑ **Who's responsible for implementation, management and evaluation?** The old saying that "where everyone's in charge, nobody's in charge" applies here. Clarifying who will lead the analysis, decision-making, implementation and operational phases is essential to project success.

❑ **How will you know whether you've succeeded or failed?**
Merely implementing a venture by moving in equipment, renovating space and the like is only one measure of success. What will the group use to evaluate the project's status? Consider evaluation criteria of a financial and operational nature. Other considerations might include practice logistics, patient and provider convenience, and quality. Identify the factors to consider in evaluating the revenue opportunity before the new venture is created. Also plan in advance how often to apply and assess the evaluation criteria.

❑ **What's the next strategy that will be required to help support the practice as a learning, growing organization?** Perhaps the only constant in health care and physician practices is that change is continual, rapid and sometimes harsh. Don't get complacent once a new strategy is implemented and well under way. While the time might not be right to move to another strategy, an ability to ask hard questions and think innovatively will likely be an essential element of a practice's long-term success.

CHAPTER 6
Conclusion

In a time of stagnant or declining reimbursement for professional services, medical groups are understandably looking for new ways to bring in additional revenues. The changing reimbursement environment encourages medical groups and their providers to think more creatively about revenue-stream diversification. In doing so, groups may now be more willing to consider strategies that involve greater levels of business complexity and/or legal risk. Recent regulatory changes in the Stark law final rule and others have opened up new opportunities.

In the face of declining reimbursement, virtually all medical groups today are trying to think differently and change their historic practices. In considering business diversification and revenue-stream enhancement strategies, practices must pay close attention to a new venture's financial and business prospects, operational demands and myriad legal and regulatory issues. While those issues can sometimes serve as barriers to a great idea, in most cases providers can develop business diversification strategies that balance their business, financial and other goals with applicable legal imperatives.

Appendixes

Appendix A. Pro Forma Income/Cash Flow Statement

Appendix B. Scorecard: Are you ready for revenue diversification?

Appendix C. Additional Resources

Appendix A. Pro Forma Income/Cash Flow Statement

Proposed Initiative _____

Year _____	Jan	Feb	Mar	Apr	May	Jun	6-Month Total	Jul	Aug	Sep	Oct	Nov	Dec	12-Month Totals	24-Month Totals	36-Month Totals
Total Services																
Gross Billings																
Collections (Revenue)																
Operating Costs																
Employee / Provider Costs																
Information Technology																
Medical / Surgical Supplies																
Building / Occupancy																
Furniture / Equipment																
Professional Liability																
Other Insurance																
Outside Professional Fees																
Promotion / Marketing																
Total Operating Costs																
Interest Expense																
Loan Payments																
Net Earnings / (Loss)																
Accumulated Earnings / (Loss)																
Accumulated Excess Cash Flow																

Appendix B. Scorecard: Are you ready for revenue diversification?

Rate your organization's preparedness for revenue diversification:	Yes	No	Uncertain
1. My group has a shared desire to grow and prosper.	3	1	2
2. My group refers a significant number of patients to other providers for ancillary services that we could provide.	3	1	2
3. Other groups or hospitals already provide the type of services my group might offer.	1	3	2
4. Other groups (or a hospital) are willing to partner in the development of new service lines.	3	1	2
5. Payers in my community will reimburse for the types of services we might provide.	3	0	2
6. My group has capital resources or reasonable access to capital necessary for the development of new business strategies.	3	1	2
7. A number of my group's physicians will retire within the next 3 to 7 years.	1	3	2
8. My group has the ability to expand facilities to accommodate new services.	3	1	2
9. My group's legal counsel specializes in health care business law and compliance.	3	1	2
10. My group understands and observes sound business behaviors.	3	1	2
11. Diversifying my group's revenue is solely intended to preserve physician incomes.	1	3	2
12. Total each column			
Sum the totals in line 12 to get your score:			

Your Score:

25 to 33 - Your group appears to have the basic qualities necessary to diversify its revenue through the delivery of new services.

20 to 34 - Your group may have the qualities necessary to diversify its revenue, but additional due diligence is necessary before delving into such activities.

10 to 19 - The desire may exist, but many of the other components of success are probably absent. Spend more time evaluating the opportunities and talking to other groups that have successfully launched new revenue strategies. Identify and address any practice weakness that might improve your score.

0 to 9 - Now is not the time to launch new services. Your group possibly lacks the unified commitment and organizational strengths required to diversify. The additional stress that such activities inherently carry could cause serious conflict among your group's members.

Appendix C. Additional Resources

Books

Ambulatory Care Management, 3rd Edition, by Austin Ross, Jr., MPH, FACMPE, Stephen J. Williams, ScD, and Ernest J. Pavlock, PhD, CPA, Delmar Publishers, 1998, available from MGMA

Assessment Manual for Medical Groups, 4th Edition by Darrell L. Schryver, DPA (editor), Medical Group Management Association, 2002

Chart of Accounts for Health Care Organizations by Neill F. Piland, DrPH, and Kathryn Glass, MBA, MSHA, MGMA Center for Research, 1999

Financial Management for Medical Groups, 2nd Edition by Ernest J. Pavlock, PhD, CPA, MGMA Center for Research, 2000

Looking for the Cashcow: Action Steps to Improve Cash Flow in Medical Group Practices by Thomas Hajny, MGMA Center for Research, 2000

Medical Practice Reimbursement Manual by Noelle Floreen, Healthcare Financial Management Association, 1998, available from MGMA

Perfect Practice for an Efficient Physician by Sherry Delio, MPA, Medical Group Management Association, 1999

Physician Compensation: Models for Aligning Financial Goals and Incentives, 2nd Edition by Kenneth M. Hekman, FACMPE, Medical Group Management Association, 2002

Rightsizing: Appropriate Staffing for your Medical Practice by Deborah Walker, MBA, FACMPE and Dave Gans, MHSA, CMPE, Medical Group Management Association, 2003

RVUs: Applications for Medical Practice Success by Kathryn P. Glass, MBA, MSHA (editor), Medical Group Management Association, 2003

Associations/Institutes

American College of Medical Practice Executives, 104 Inverness Terrace East, Englewood, CO, 80112, 877-275-6462, www.mgma.com/acmpe

American College of Physician Executives, 4890 West Kennedy Boulevard, Suite 200, Tampa, FL 33609, 800-562-8088, www.acpe.org

American Medical Group Association, 1422 Duke Street, Alexandria, VA 22314, 703-838-0033, www.amga.org

American Medical Association, 515 North State Street, Chicago, IL 60610, 312-464-5000, www.ama-assn.org

American Medical Informatics Association, 4915 St. Elmo Avenue, Suite 401, Bethesda, MD 20814, 301-657-1291, www.amia.org

Healthcare Financial Management Association, Two Westbrook Corporate Center, Suite 700, Westchester, IL 60154-5700, 800-252-HFMA, www.hfma.org

Medical Group Management Association, 104 Inverness Terrace East, Englewood, CO, 80112, 877-ASK-MGMA, www.mgma.com

Specialty Societies and Associations (complete listing found at www.ama-assn.org)

State Medical Societies (complete listing found at www.ama-assn.org)

Benchmarking

MGMA *Coding Profile Sourcebook*

MGMA *Cost Survey Report*

MGMA *Management Compensation Survey Report*

MGMA *Performance and Practices of Successful Medical Groups*

MGMA *Physician Compensation and Production Survey*

Physcape[SM] *Inc.* (MGMA Services, Inc.)

Physician Socioeconomic Statistics (AMA)

Index

T

V

W

Z